Menopause:

7 secret ways on How you can overcome it, feel young again, and regain your confidence.

```
I0411129
```

By Julie Clark

Table of Contents

Chapter 1: Understanding Menopause

Menopause—a word feared by many women.

Over time, the word menopause became associated with a lot of negativity. Some may look at it as the beginning of the end as it often signifies the end of a woman's child bearing years. It is not uncommon for some women to feel a sense of worthlessness in knowing that their ability to reproduce is over. Some may feel a sense of loss. Others look at it as a phase in life that is full of hot flashes, bone loss, and just an overall decline in health. It is a dreary and very unappealing life to look forward to.

Many women go through their menopause years clueless on what will happen, how it will happen, and how long it will last. They just woke up one day feeling that something is not right with their bodies. Because of these, they often find themselves scared, confused, and apprehensive.

They have no idea what is happening to them. They feel lost and alone, thinking that something is wrong with their bodies.

Understanding what menopause is all about will help appease these fears. It is not a disease or condition that needs to be cured. It is a natural stage in life that every woman will go through. No one can control it. It is something that is inevitable. Knowing why it happens and how it happens will help women deal with this new stage in their lives in the most effective way possible. It will show them how they can continue to enjoy their prime years while managing the symptoms and signs of reaching menopause.

Menopause is not the end. It is in fact the beginning of a new phase in their lives. Knowledge and understanding will liberate them and give them the freedom to enjoy the next chapter in their lives.

To understand menopause, it is important to start with the basics.

The word menopause itself literally means the "end of the cycles "from the root word *men* (month) and the Greek word *pausis* which means cessation. The word describes a stage in a woman's life when menstruation stops permanently, thus marking the end of her ability to reproduce.

Menopause is the opposite of menarche. Menarche defines the stage in a young woman's life when menstruation begins. Her ovaries start producing eggs. At this point in her life, she becomes capable of bearing children. During menopause, a woman's ovaries are considered officially out of business. They will cease operations and become inactive. It is scientifically defined as the absence of menstrual flow or periods and this will happen once the ovaries themselves have stopped their primary functions.

The ovaries are the core parts of a woman's reproductive system. She has two of these almond-shaped glands. Each month, an ovary produces an egg or ovum. These ovaries are also responsible for producing hormones which in turn, causes the walls of the uterus to thicken, ideally preparing it for implantation of a fertilized egg. If fertilization does not happen, the uterus will later on shed or discard the uterine lining. These are the menses or period that a woman experiences each month. When menopause occurs, all of these activities inside a woman's body will stop permanently.

The common misconception of menopause is that it happens at a certain age or year in woman's life. This is not necessarily the case. It is a natural phase in a woman's life and just like any phase in life, it is also made up of several stages. The transition from the reproductive state to being non-reproductive is a gradual process. It is not something that happens over night. It occurs over a certain number of years. It starts around late 40s or early 50s and may go on for a few more years or even a decade.

There are four stages of menopause that a woman will go through. Knowing when they will happen will help women brace themselves in facing the years leading up to menopause and the years after that: **Premenopausal** This is the term used to describe the years leading up to the last menstruation. This happens around mid to late 40s. There might be no glaring symptoms yet but at this point, the levels of reproductive hormones are beginning to wane.

Perimenopause This term refers to the transition years to menopause. The events that happen and the changes that occur in their bodies during these years are often incorrectly associated with the term menopause.

The word's literal meaning is "around menopause." This is often considered as the dreaded stage. The North American Menopause Society estimates that this stage can last for four to eight years while The Centre for Menstrual Cycle and Ovulation Research said that it can last up to ten years!

At this point, hormone levels become erratic. There are high points, like estrogen levels reaching by more than 20% to 30%, and there are also low points when hormones levels drop significantly. These fluctuations will often manifest physically. This is when a woman begins to experience the infamous symptoms of what they often thought of as "menopause." The more accurate term to use is actually the perimenopause phase.

Some of these symptoms are hot flashes, vaginal dryness, mood swings, sweating, palpitations, decreased libido, osteoporosis or bone loss, and trouble sleeping (These symptoms and their management will be tackled in detail in the later chapters.).

Though some may feel the signs of the transition phase as early as age 35, most symptoms become evident once a woman hits her late 40s. And since this stage can last up to ten years, a woman's body will go through a lot of changes as her body continues to adjust to the constant up and down of hormones.

Menopause This stage is clinically defined as the date exactly twelve months after a woman last had her menstrual flow. At this point, the ovaries have officially ceased their functions. They have stopped producing eggs and most of the estrogen in the body.

Postmenopause This stage pretty much comprises the years ahead, after one year of no menstrual period at all or menopause. As the level of reproductive hormones continues to drop (until the ovaries become inactive), the occurrences of the dreaded symptoms also start to go away. Any spotting or bleeding that may occur during these years is not normal and should be brought to a doctor's attention right away.

How can you be sure, you are experiencing menopause? Let us look at menopause symptoms.

Hot flashes, night sweats, and insomnia

Hot flashes are probably the very first menopausal symptom you'll experience. Most women approaching menopause (premenopausal) experience hot flashes that usually last 2-4 minutes. You usually suddenly start feeling heat from your face spreading to your upper body and then all over, with a bit of sweating and blushing, often followed by chills and shivers as your body tries to regulate temperatures. Some women have severe hot flashes while others mild with some experiencing them while still having their periods while others when their menses stop. It's not yet known why hot flashes occur but scientists feel the core of this problem is in the hypothalamus (base of the brain) and the brains thermoregulatory center as they try to react to estrogen withdrawal.

You may have hot flashes every hour of the day/night or once after a couple of days. Hot flashes are often associated with insomnia and heart palpitations. Estrogen boosts serotonin; a chemical that helps you sleep and prevents depression plus increasing GABA (brain stuff that makes you feel calm and good), while progesterone helps balance estrogen. Therefore, abnormal progesterone levels, cause insomnia and mood imbalances.

Unsurprisingly, women with intense sleep disturbances are normally moody and grouchy the following day. When hot flashes occur frequently during the day you may feel uncomfortable and embarrassed while at night you may have unrelenting insomnia, which could lead to irritability, fatigue, depression, anxiety, and concentration problems (may even lose focus on job-related tasks). These symptoms are more linked to chronic sleep disturbances than menopause in itself.

You may occasionally experience hot flashes during premenopausal phase-don't take this as a sign of an imminent menopause though. Some of us will have hot flashes for more than a year-if untreated they last for a few years but some (5-

10%) women will have them past 70. Obese women are more prone to hot flashes as well as women who smoke and live a sedentary lifestyle.

Irregular or skipped periods

You will experience many changes in your normal menses. As you approach menopause, production of progesterone and estrogen declines and ovulation stops. This decline in progesterone shortens your cycle length (count from the first day you get your menses to the first day of your next period). For instance, a cycle length of usually 27-30 days may reduce to 22-26 days and, as your menses become somehow irregular, with 'cycles' differing by three to five weeks apart, declining progesterone may also shorten your period-. Your menses may last for fewer days and even get lighter or heavier. Some women may start spotting before their normal menstrual flow begins. All these changes are due to the falling levels of progesterone and estrogen. As menopause progresses, you could even skip a period but, test to confirm you aren't pregnant.

Urinary inconsistency/bladder control issues

Urinary inconsistency is rather common among menopausal women which makes you find it hard to hold your urine long enough to reach the bathroom. You may suddenly get an urge to urinate or your urine could leek during exercise, coughing or sneezing. It normally starts or worsens during premenopausal because the bladder tissues and its supporting structure depend on estrogen.

Low sex drive

Lose of sexual energy during premenopausal and menopausal phase is a complicated phenomenon that may or may not be linked to the simple hormonal changes. Besides the loss of estrogen, there is loss of testosterone (another hormone made by ovaries) which plays a key role in sexual desire. Quite a number of things could cause you to lose your sexual energy, such as, depression, low energy levels, and family or work pressure and complicated relationship with your sexual partner. Many women who have experienced very satisfying sex well into their 40s and 50s who suddenly lose interest in sex. However, you could also feel much freer and sexier after menopause-after all you can't get pregnant but, watch out for STDs.

Vaginal dryness and atrophy

Low estrogen causes a decrease in blood flow to the vagina and vulva and reduces the amount and quality of vaginal lubrication. In the cause of time the vagina suffers degenerative changes (atrophy) that make your vaginal wall shorter and narrower especially you've not had sex for years. Generally, atrophy develops 5-10 years after the start of menopausal hot flashes. Moreover, the vagina dries because its lining is not making enough mucus. The urethra (bladder outlet tube) also experience similar changes. This may cause urinary tract infections (UTIs) due to bacteria overgrowth.

Additional symptoms

Thinning hair, itching under skin, short-term memory loss, reduced breast size, joint and muscle aches, and headaches can also occur due to estrogen loss among other reasons like aging.

However, since we're different not all of us experience all these symptoms. In fact, some women don't have hot flashes as their first symptom.

Long-Term Health Problems Related to Menopause

Since your estrogen levels dwindle during menopause, you may start experiencing a number of health problems.

After menopause, you may suffer from conditions such as:

Osteoporosis

Your body is always crashing old bones and replacing them with new healthy bones. Estrogen aids in regulating bone lose and when you lose estrogen during menopause, you lose more bone than is replaced. Therefore, your bones may become weak and fragile leading to a condition known as osteoporosis. Consult your doctor to see if you are at risk and seek treatment. Also, use the bone health tips I'll offer later.

Malfunctioning bladder and bowel

Pelvic floor muscles weaken due to lose of estrogen. Because these muscles control your bladder and bowel, their weakness may reduce your ability to hold or control your urge to visit the toilet. In addition, your bladder could lose elasticity causing frequent urination and significant weight gain can further weaken your pelvic muscle worsening this situation.

Increased wrinkling

Hormonal changes affect skin physiology. This is because estrogen stimulates fat deposits, which are then redistributed and stored in our abdomen, thighs and buttocks. Consequently, we lose the supportive fats in our face, neck, arms and hands causing sagging and wrinkles. Moreover, your breast may lose fat deposits causing them to sag and flatten.

Heart disease

After menopause, women are prone to heart disease due to changes in estrogen levels and aging. Age could come with possible weight gain (our body stores fat so it becomes harder for you to lose weight) and other problems like high blood pressure, which put you at risk of heart disease.

Eye problems

Hormonal changes during menopause can cause vision problems and even cataracts.

Now that you have all the basics about menopause, let's look at a number of simple effective ideas to help you cope with the troubling menopausal symptoms and lower the risks associated with these serious post-menopausal conditions.

How to Deal with Menopause Symptoms

Let us look at how to deal with menopause symptoms by learning how to take care of your adrenal glands.

Take Care of Your Adrenal Glands During Menopause

Poor glandular function is a major contributor to your hot flushes and sleepless nights. When our ovaries stop making, progesterone, estrogen and testosterone, the adrenal glands and fat cells take over. The adrenal glands are located right above your kidneys and they produce hormones that help us deal with stress among other bodily functions. Therefore, for a very busy woman, the adrenal glands work at full capacity and to load them with the extra work of producing more hormones is the last straw. That's why many women suffer from hot flashes when going through stress.

Top foods and herbs for good adrenal health include:

Take foods rich in vitamin C

Compounds in vitamin C (bioflavonoids) have been shown to reduce hot flashes and help skin elasticity by increasing collagen, which can help with bladder problems and vaginal dryness.

Foods rich in vitamin C are citrus fruits, strawberries, tomatoes, cabbage, broccoli, kiwi fruit, rock melon, and sweet red peppers.

Take foods rich in vitamin B5 and B6

These vitamins have compounds that help ease stress on adrenal glands.

Foods rich in vitamin B5 and B6 are soybeans, brewer's yeast, sunflower seeds, eggs, avocado, and fish.

You can also support your adrenal glands using amazing herbs such as:

Ginseng

Ginseng is also known as an adaptagen because it helps the body adjust to stress. Ginseng works by increasing dopamine and serotonin, which is your brain's 'feel good' chemicals boosting your moods and sleep. In addition, it is energizing; thus, it is good to take the morning after a sleepless night with a busy day ahead. The recommended ginseng dose is 800mg to 2 g a day. It's advisable that you take ginseng with food to prevent nausea that occurs when taken on empty stomach. However, avoid taking it in excess or for more than 3months.

Withania (ashwagandha)

In addition to being an adaptagen, it reduces cortisol (which causes stress). It is also relaxing as well as a powerful aphrodisiac (boosts sex). Recommended dose of 500 to 100mg twice or thrice a day (however follow instructions on the supplement). It is advisable to take the herb at night and in the morning.

Licorice root

The special acids in licorice root help nourish the adrenal glands relieving depression and nervousness.

Sage

Sage is a phytoestrogen that also helps reduce sweating and hot flushes. It is often taken as tea.

Take phytoestrogens (plant estrogens)

Phytoestrogen are nutrients that naturally occur in plants that act similar to estrogen in our bodies. Phytoestrogens work by binding to the estrogen receptors in our cells helping to balance hormones and this in turn helps in reducing hormonal symptoms. Phytoestrogens work by also slowing cell growth and preventing inflammation. If you're one of the many women out there who dread the health risks of synthetic hormones used in the usual hormone therapies, consider phytoestrogens as an alternative. Here are its main sources:

Phytoestrogen foods

Foods rich in phytoestrogen are flax seeds and other oil seeds, soybeans, fermented soya milk and flour, peas, lentils, tofu, pumpkin seeds, nuts, fennel, apples, parsley, celery, alfalfa and whole grains especially millet and rye.

Phytoestrogen herbs

Some popular herbs that are considered phytoestrogens include; Black cohosh, Red clover, and licorice root.

We should probably borrow from our Asian sisters who evidently have fewer incidences of osteoporosis, heart disease, and cancers of the colon breast and womb, due to consuming diets rich in phytoestrogen. In addition, these women apparently don't get serious hot flashes and night sweats like their western counter parts.

Therefore, when you consume a diet rich in phytoestrogen you get various health benefits including relief from menopausal symptoms and less risk of the so-called "western diseases". Therefore, take large amounts of phytoestrogen in foods or herbal supplements (remember to consult your doctor first).

Care for Your Liver

Looking after your liver is another key aspect in hormonal health, especially during menopause. There are several ways the liver is linked to hormonal health. First, it helps to process and distribute hormones into your blood stream where they perform their tasks of sending signals to your body and tissues. Secondly, it assists in eliminating excess hormones from the bloodstream and ships them to be expelled from your body. Therefore, it's quite involved in hormonal balance. However, if you overload your liver with too much detoxification tasks it may not work at its best, which can worsen menopausal symptoms. Therefore, if you don't want to overwork your liver quit coffee, cigarettes and alcohol (stimulants), as they trigger hot flashes. Take healthy alternatives like water or green tea instead. Cut out sugar, junk food and avoid environmental chemicals (e.g. chemical cleaning products, sprays, fumes etc.), since most packaged foods may contain chemicals that overburden your liver.

Then support your liver function by taking plenty of water (at least 8 glasses a day), and give it antioxidants to help in the cleansing process. Fruits and vegetables are rich in antioxidants.

In addition, many herbs support the liver, the major ones being milk thistle and globe artichoke.

Your Blood Sugar Levels and Menopause

Balanced blood sugar levels highly depend on what you eat or don't eat. When you eat sugary foods and simple carbohydrates, they are quickly digested and converted into glucose, which causes sharp spikes to your blood sugar levels, which is often followed by a sharp dip that can leave you feeling tired, grumpy, and craving for starchier or sugary snacks that only worsen your situation. In addition, the excess glucose is stored as fats or converted to energy.

It is important to note that sudden rise and fall of sugar levels has been shown to cause many other problems in the body. Apart from causing weight gain, taking refined carbs and sugars can also be the root cause of your agonizing periods and menopause symptoms. Cutting down on refined sugar and carbs has been shown to reduce some menopausal symptoms like irritability and mood swings. Sugar not only causes major highs and lows in energy and mood but, it also disrupts insulin, a hormone that is closely linked to all hormones in your body including testosterone and estrogen and also helps keep the blood sugar at normal levels. Therefore, balancing your blood sugar can really help stabilize your energy and moods.

Here are some simple ideas that can help prevent blood sugar imbalances:

Eat a healthy breakfast

Start your day with veggie-protein rich breakfast. Missing your breakfast will destabilize your energy and mood levels.

Eat less but often

We need fewer calories as we age. In addition to cutting back on sugar, watch the fat in your diet. Only eat unsaturated fats found in lean meats, wild fish and vegetable oils (olive, coconut etc.). Take 5-6 small portions of food per day to have energy throughout your day (three modest meals and 2 healthy snacks will do). Also, ensure that your plate has more veggies than carbs.

Include protein in each meal

Proteins have slower energy release, which ensures you don't experience blood sugar spikes. Great protein sources include foods such as meat, eggs, legumes, nuts and dairy. The solution is variety and good combination of protein and energy sources.

Eat Foods high in fiber

Fiber is found in almost all fresh vegetables and fruits especially asparagus, collard greens, eggplant, broccoli, turnips, squash, and beets. Whole grains like whole wheat, brown rice, sorghum, barley, oats and pseudo grains such as quinoa and spelt are also full of fiber. Take these foods because fiber takes time to digest and this in turn keeps your blood sugar stable. In addition, they keep you fuller for longer so won't have the cravings.

Minimize or rather cut off foods such as white rice, white bread, white pasta and all other white flour products which have practically zero fiber causing blood sugar imbalances.

Protect Your Bones

Your bone density starts decreasing during menopause. Therefore, increase your intake of minerals like magnesium, Calcium, and nutrients like vitamins D and K to maintain your bone density. Let us see how these minerals and nutrients help with menopause.

Magnesium

Magncsium helps with mood swings, anxiety and irritability as well as bone strength. Foods rich in magnesium include leafy green veggies, nuts, seeds, kelp, oyster, shrimp, and avocados.

Vitamin D

It assists in absorption of calcium and vitamin K and limits osteoporosis and type-2 diabetes. Low levels of vitamin D are linked to bowel disease, poor immune function among other things. Just bask 15 minutes a day under morning or late afternoon sun to get your dose of vitamin D or, take vitamin D supplements.

Consider taking other vitamins and minerals necessary for healthy bones such as vitamin E (also good for vaginal dryness and flushes) and zinc. Opt for a supplement that has a combination of minerals and vitamins.

Avoid foods high in phosphorous

Phosphorous is found in food such as; red meat, processed food as well as fizzy drinks. Phosphorous is not good because too much phosphorus in your diet speeds up the loss of minerals such as magnesium and calcium from your bones. Reducing sodium (salt), animal protein, and caffeine can enhance calcium storage.

Choose alkaline foods

Take plenty of fruits vegetables, seeds, nuts and unsweetened yoghurt to help prevent lose of calcium from your bones.

Eat foods high in magnesium and boron

These minerals are essential for bone replacement thus helping lower your risk of osteoporosis. Good sources of boron are pears, apples, grapes, raisins and dates.

Do weight bearing exercise

You should work those muscles and keep your bone sturdy. I'll talk more about this in the exercise section.

Get Adequate Sleep

When it comes to sleep, quality matters more than quantity. What you feel when you wake up tells a lot about how you slept. Often the cure to your sleep difficulties and daytime fatigue is found in your lifestyle choices and daily routine.

Here are some ideas that you can experiment with to sleep better:

Optimize your bedroom environment

The first step is to make your bedroom an optimized ideal environment for sleeping. Here is how:

*Plug your phone charger in an outlet far away from your bed to avoid grabbing your phone while lying down. Doing this stopped me from watching You Tube or checking Facebook before I fell asleep. In fact, watching bright screens 1-2 hours before bedtime disrupts sleep.

*Wear a sleeping mask and keep the curtains drawn to make your room as dark as possible. Once your room is full optimized, set your reminder for bedtime.

Commit to a consistent bedtime and wakeup time

Try to go to sleep and wake up at the same time each day. Doing this helps reset your body's internal clock and optimizes your sleep's quality. Pick a bedtime when you're really tired to avoid tossing and turning. Prepare some minutes before your bedtime and then when the time comes, switch off the light, close your eyes, focus on your breath rhythms and let sleep take over you.

Take smart naps

A critical aspect in dealing with menopausal symptoms such as anxiety and all other sleep-related symptoms is taking a 20-minute nap every early afternoon. Longer naps can interfere with your sleep at night. After you've had lunch, take a nap. Set 20-minute alarm on your phone, lie on your back with your eyes shut. Don't try so much to fall asleep, instead focus on breathing in and out. Even if you don't fall asleep you'll feel refreshed and calm every time after your alarm goes off.

Fight after-dinner drowsiness

If you feel sleepy way ahead of your set bedtime, get up and wash the dishes, call a friend or prepare clothes for the next day or anything else mildly stimulating.

Drink warm milk

Warm milk is an ancient remedy for insomnia. A glass of milk anytime of the day helps tame tension. This is because milk contains an amino acid known as tryptophan, which aids in production of serotonin which s your mood and promotes your well-being.

Next, I'll cover relaxation techniques that you can do before bed to help you sleep better among other things.

Effective Relaxation Techniques

Sometimes we are so caught up in our lives that we've no time for relaxation. Getting enough rest will lessen menopausal symptoms such as anxiety, stress, and insomnia among others. Take some time to calm your mind using any of the following techniques:

Deep breathing

1. Lie on your back keeping your body relaxed. Place your hands on your stomach and close your eyes.

2. Take deep slow breaths in and out and make each breath deeper than the previous.

3. Continue doing this until you fall asleep.

Doing this for just 5 minutes will significantly affect your heart rate and blood pressure.

Progressive muscle relation

Lie on your back with your eyes closed. Tense your toes as tightly as possible release after 10 seconds. Tense the rest of your muscles. Work your way up to your knees, thighs, stomach, chest, buttocks, cheeks, hands and finally roll your shoulders around. Relax after you work on each muscle.

Visual imagery

Visualize a serene restful place. Close your eyes and start Imagining a calming place or activity. Focus on how relaxed this place makes you feel. Go back there whenever necessary. Visiting this place more and more will help you fall asleep easier.

Yoga

Yoga is a powerful antidote for insomnia and stress. Research has proven that if done regularly, yoga lessens menopausal symptoms. You can take a yoga class but here is a simple pose to help you wind down:

Corpse pose

Do the following:

Lie on your back. Slightly stretch out your arm and legs. Rest your palms on the floor. Think of good and positive things. Stretch out any tension in your limbs. Imagine that you're so heavy and being supported by the floor. Do this for around 5 minutes.

Medication

Another great way of dealing with your everyday stress and getting quality sleep is meditation.

Try this:

1. Find a quiet place and sit on a chair with your back straight.

2. Put one hand on your abdomen.

3. Concentrate on your lung sensations as you breathe in through your nose and out through your mouth.

4. Feel your stomach rise and fall beneath your hand. Do this for 10 minutes.

This will help clear any worries in your mind.

Massage

Massage is an old healing trick that still does wonders. With a regular massage you' feel calm and deeply relaxed even way after your massage is over. Consider having aromatherapy massage (uses essential oils).

Take a little chocolate

Taking loads of chocolate for relaxation is a universal truth. When you take chocolate your brain muscles relax and this helps reduce anxiety and stress. Choose organic raw unsweetened chocolate and bite occasionally during the day to keep your sugar level stable.

Use lavender

This amazing anti-inflammatory herb relaxes your cells and reduces mind inflammation and this helps with, stress and anxiety.

1. Fill an infuser with lavender oil and put in your room or buy lavender fragrance and spray it in your room or keep a bottle of it nearby.

2. Wear a lotion scented with lavender or take lavender pills

Exercise

Daily vigorous physical activity has been proven to relieve stress as well as ease menopausal symptoms such as hot flushes and night sweats, improve sleep and balance hormones. In addition, regular exercise limits loss of muscle mass and weight gain, which are common side effects of menopause. The center for disease control (CDC) agrees that a healthy woman should have a minimum of 150 minutes of moderate physical activity a week.

Here are some effective exercise ideas you can consider:

Cardio

An aerobic activity that utilizes your larger muscle groups and maintains your heart rate is a win. You have no limit for cardio as jogging, walking, biking, and swimming are all considered as weight bearing exercises. As a newbie consider starting with 10 minutes of light activity then slowly increase your work out intensity to at least 20 minutes a day as it become easier.

Strength training

This workout minimizes your risk of osteoporosis and other bone problems. These exercises are vital because they'll help in building your bone and muscle strength, boosting your metabolism and burning body fat.

While at home, opt for resistance tubing and dumbbells. In the gym, either free weights or weight machines will do. Choose a level hard enough to tax your muscles in about 12 repetitions then gradually increase your intensity.

Dancing

Who said exercise can't be fun! Having a calories burning session in your routine is fun and good for you. If you do prefer running on the treadmill, then consider taking a dance class. Dancing keeps you flexible and builds muscle.

You can even dance to your favorite music in your bedroom.

Vigorous chores

Vigorous house/yard work that increases your heart rate and uses your larger muscle groups like, glutes, squads, and core work wonders (halfhearted dusting doesn't count). For a beginner, you can start with 10 minutes of light activity then go from there. Sweep, trim fences, mow the lawn, or do any other relevant thing you can think of.

Use Essential Oils

Essential oils (liquid plant extracts) have healing properties. They can be beneficial during menopause owing to their soothing, harmonizing and balancing effects on the mind. For instance, sage oil is the most effective essential oil for relief from menopausal symptoms like hot flashes. Furthermore, Roman chamomile oil reduces stress while peppermint oil can help in cooling your body from hot flashes.

I recommend the following oils for menopause; sage, roman chamomile, geranium, rose, lavender, peppermint and thyme

How to use

Vaporize; Add 6-9 drops of preferred essential oil to water inside the top of your vaporizer.

Body rubs: To reconnect with your femininity do this 'ritual' daily. Add 6 drops of your preferred essential oil to 12 ml jojoba oils. Apply to your body in circular motions. Start from your feet and work your way up towards your neck

Aromatic tissue: Add 1-3 drops to a tissue or cotton ball then inhale.

In bath water: Add 6 drops of preferred essential oil to a teaspoon of sweet almond before you put in your warm bath water.

Ingest: Soak sage in lemon juice and take two teaspoonsful before bedtime to fight the night sweats. Seek advice from an expert before ingesting any essential oil.

Note; Test if you're sensitive to essential on a soft part of your hand plus always dilute with a vegetable oil (such as sweet almond, coconut oil, olive oil...) to avoid skin reaction.

Chapter 2: Natural Remedies for Menopause

For centuries, women from all over the world have learned to deal with the symptoms of menopause. Even in recent years, menopausal women choose to deal with their condition in a natural approach. Menopause can be dealt with without medications and if you would rather conquer the problem this way, you should consider the following herbs and supplements: First consult your doctor before taking any supplements.

- Flaxseed (Linum usitassimum): Whether you enjoy flaxseed or flaxseed oil, it can help deal with mild menopause symptoms. About 1.5 ounces or (40 grams) of ground flaxseed per day is enough to reduce the overall effect of hot flashes. With prolonged use, you can see a significant decrease in the frequency and intensity of hot flashes, by 50%.

Flaxseed contains a very good source of lignan, a powerful antioxidant that can fight against cancer; and also contains a good amount of omega-3 fatty acids which will provide necessary protection against heart disease. Apart from hot flashes and night sweats, flaxseed is also found to be good for muscle pain and mood improvement.

- Vitamin E: As early as the 1940s, scientific studies have shown that Vitamin E has the capacity to reduce the effects of hot flashes to 50%. As long as you maintain the dosage below 400 international units (IU), taking vitamin E will be safe and will not cause any dangerous side effects.

Apart from hot flashes, Vitamin E is also an amazing help for night sweats, palpitations and a range of heart problems. Talk to your doctor first before taking vitamin E supplements: It is dangerous when taken in high quantities.

- Omega 3's: Fish are rich in Omega 3-fatty acids, the healthy type of fat that your body needs a lot of to stay healthy. As a rule, you should enjoy at least two portions of oily fish a week such as fresh tuna, salmon, mackerel and sardines to provide the body with enough good fat that will protect your tissues and organs. Omega 3's also reduce inflammation and improve bone density in women who are menopausal.

- Red Clover: Red clover contains high levels of isoflavones, water-soluble compounds that act like estrogen. This type of plant is a phytoestrogen that is rich in various vitamins and minerals (Vitamin C, thiamine, chromium, calcium, potassium, phosphorus, niacin, magnesium and phosphorus) that has the capacity to deal with menopausal symptoms such as hot flashes, osteoporosis and reduce the chances of developing endometrial cancer.

Side Affects: some caution must be taken, however, because some cases revealed that the use of red clover for over 3 months can increase the risk of developing uterine cancer.

- Fiber: There is bloating and weight gain related to menopause. Fiber from fruits, vegetables, oats, lentils and beans will help cleanse your body, control your weight and keep your digestive tract healthy.

Fiber contains a generous amount of cellulose that cannot be digested by human beings. When eaten, fiber can curb the appetite and control cholesterol levels by attaching to fat so that it may be flushed out of the body as waste material.

- St. John's Wort: Depression is a common symptom of menopause, due to the drastic changes going on with in a woman's body. St. John's Wort (SJW) is a known treatment for mild cases of depression and there is also proof of its capacity to enhance a woman's sex drive.

Note: When combined with black cohosh its efficacy will be even more appreciated.

- Black Cohosh: Quite popular in Europe, Black Cohosh, is the most well-studied supplement for menopause, it is a herbal supplement that can help treat hot flashes. It is made from the root of the North American black cohosh plant and is an ideal treatment because it can be taken for up to 1 year. Unfortunately, studies have shown that prolonged use of black cohosh stops showing effects after 6 months to a year. But this would be a great way to help your body deal with the beginning stages of menopause.

- Vitamin D: Vitamin D is required for strong bones. You can either go in the sun for about 15 minutes per day or incorporate more Vitamin D-rich foods into your diet, so that you can prevent any skeletal complications related to menopause. Adults need about 600 IU of Vitamin D on a daily basis.

Apart from all that, Vitamin D helps prevent heart disease, weight gain, depression and cancer: a. osteoporosis: In combination with calcium, Vitamin D can help strengthen the bones that become weaker due to age and exacerbated by menopause.

b. depression: Vitamin D is good for mood and cognitive performance. Since extreme mood changes often lead to depression, a little boost with the help of Vitamin D is going to be of value.

c. cancer: With the right dose, Vitamin D can suppress the growth of malignant cancers that may have developed during the time of menopause.

d. heart disease: The decrease in estrogen levels often increase the risk of developing heart disease. Equipping yourself with vitamin D is going to be help your body cope with this change.

- Wild Yams: Yams contain a considerable amount of estrogen and progesterone, so they are very good for women and their menstrual cycle. Similarly, its benefits extend up to their menopausal age. It is for this reason that wild yams are often found in pills and creams that are used to treat menopause symptoms.

- Soy: Soy has been found to be good for menopausal women for various reasons: a. It contains isoflavones that can mimic the action of natural estrogen in the body b. It helps control the hormonal fluctuations that usually occur in menopausal women c. It can reduce the effect symptoms—reducing the intensity and frequency of hot flashes and controlling weight gain.

d. It is rich in calcium, so it can help prevent osteoporosis and it can also prevent the development of breast cancer by properly maintaining the equilibrium of the hormones in the body e. It is an excellent source of iron so it can help boost energy

Soy can be enjoyed in form of soy nuts and tofu—and as long as it is taken in regulation can really do wonders. As a matter of fact, theories are circulating that since women from Asia feature soy as a staple, it can explain why hot flashes are a greater issue with women from America than those from Asia.

- Ginseng: For many centuries, ginseng has been a powerful natural pharmaceutical. Its capacity to prevent various complications make it a very good companion for menopause. Ginseng is a good helper during menopause because it can help improve sleeping habits and it can improve your mood. Ginseng can help with hot flashes because it will lower your body temperature, and therefore relieve episodes of hot flashes.

-Calcium: Many women who reach menopause develop all kinds of skeletal problems such as osteoporosis. The bones become weak due to hormone decline and the intake of calcium cam help make your bones stronger. You can either add more calcium to your diet or take calcium tablets.

Note: calcium supplements should be taken 500 milligrams at a time and not all in one go. If you are enjoying your calcium dosage through your diet, this should not be an issue. Cutting down the dosage to 500 milligrams at a time will make it easier to absorb. (Speak to your doctor before taking calcium supplements.)

- Dong Quai: Popular in China for years, it has been very popular for treating various health issues. For menopause, dong quai has been trusted for hot flashes, but its use should be controlled since it can bring various risks, including cancer.

Planning a diet that is rich in essential vitamins and minerals will help make a potentially awful experience, somewhat bearable. It may not solve the issue, completely, but it will bring you some relief. Apart from your diet, it is also smart to generously hydrate your body with water. Consuming at least 8 glasses a day will be very good for cleansing, lubrication and hydration. This will also help relieve symptoms like hot flashes and vaginal dryness.

Again, it is important to research and consult with your doctor about any supplements or medications you are taking and how they may interact with one another. Ask your doctor before you start taking any supplements.

Hormones play a big part during menopause. They explain a lot why women experience a lot of changes in their bodies during menopause. They are the reasons behind those often awful symptoms and discomforts women go through during the perimenopause stage. Understanding what they are and how they work will give women a better understanding of the changes that are happening inside their bodies.

Hormones are defined as chemicals that are naturally secreted by various glands in a human body. These chemical secretions travel all over the blood stream from one body organ to another. They are considered the body's messengers as they communicate with the different parts of the body and affect the different processes in the body like growth, metabolism, reproduction and even moods and emotions. Too little or too much of these hormones are always not a good thing and may cause unwanted changes in the body.

The ovaries are the focus glands in this chapter. This is because they are the glands responsible for producing the hormones that play crucial roles during menopause.

Ovaries are a tiny pair of glands shaped like almonds and are located on opposite sides of the uterus, in the female pelvic cavity. They produce the female sex hormones estrogen and progesterone and all throughout the years after menarche up until puberty, a woman will experience an ebb and flow of these hormones. Estrogen is considered the more dominant hormone.

Estrogen and Progesterone During puberty, estrogen is the hormone liable for the development of a woman's mammary glands or breasts tissues and her uterus. During the menstrual cycle, this hormone develops the uterine lining. During the menstrual cycle, as the estrogen surges, the menses stop, the uterine lining thickens, and the follicles in the ovary begin to develop, from which an ovum or egg is eventually released in a process called ovulation. Progesterone, on the other hand, which is produced upon ovulation, prepares the uterus for the likelihood of pregnancy as well as the mammary glands for possible lactation. Together, these two hormones work hand in hand during the menstrual cycle. If the egg is not fertilized and no implantation occurs after about two weeks, the levels of these hormones drop and cause the uterus to shed its unused lining. The shedding process is the monthly period that a woman experiences each month.

While these two hormones are commonly associated with the reproductive system, it is important to know that they also play crucial roles in other parts of the body. Estrogen for example is also responsible for calcium absorption which leads to stronger bones. It also plays a role in a woman's bladder and urethral health.

The body is working continuously to balance these hormones but certain factors, both internal and external, can cause changes in the levels of these hormones. When this happens, the body will try to cope with the changes and this is often manifested by various physical symptoms. Some factors that can alter the balance of hormones in the body are stress, medication, and change in body weight, pregnancy and menopause. Though majority of these factors are temporary in nature, menopause on the other hand, is not. It brings about permanent change in the body's hormone levels. When a woman reaches the menopause phase, her ovaries will stop producing eggs. And when that happens, they will also shut off production of estrogen and progesterone.

When a woman reaches her late 30s, her body starts to produce less progesterone. This is made apparent by heavier flows during periods. However, most of the physical signs and symptoms will show when the body's production of estrogen starts to diminish. It is at this point that the body experiences the discomforts that are often associated with the perimenopause phase.

Chapter 3: Changing Your Lifestyle

Your lifestyle can affect the intensity of the symptoms of menopause. Menopausal woman will benefit from staying active, because they will be able to deal with the symptoms associated with menopause more easily. The following are some of things you can do which have scientific significance. An even more natural approach to the condition that takes away the need for medicines and treatments will involve making a lifestyle change and incorporating these activities into your daily routine.

Here is a list of some activities and habits you can incorporate into your everyday life:

- Exercises: It does not matter type of exercising you do; it will help make your life better as you go through the stages of menopause. Exercising will strengthen your cardiovascular system, improve your mood by releasing endorphins, protect your body against diabetes, as well as osteoporosis by strengthen your bones and muscles.

If you have been an avid health buff throughout your life continue your normal routine even into your menopausal years. If you have never done any exercising through out your life, do not be threatened to start a new routine because it will be easy to get used to the activity once you get your groove and find a specific exercise you enjoy. There a number of different activities you can do: running, biking, dancing, swimming, aerobics and so many others. To find which on is best for you, try many different things until you find the activities you enjoy doing. When you find an exercise that is right for you commit to a regular routine so that you can truly see the great health benefits you will get from a consistent effort.

- Yoga: Yoga is not only a physical exercise it is an activity that can condition your mind as well. When you participate in yoga, you are able to increase your flexibility and you develop stronger muscles and bones in the process. Also, the meditative nature of yoga will help you deal with the mood swings associated with menopause. Menopausal women are easily irritated and annoyed so meditation will help to calm the nerves and ease the tension. A healthy mind and body is what you will get when you practice yoga. There are many different types of yoga classes you can join at your gym. Try them all until you find the one you like. You can also find exercise videos online that you can do at home, at youtube.com or you can purchase exercise dvds as well.

- Breathing Exercises: You will learn deep breathing techniques through your yoga instructor. Deep breathing is a very effective relaxation technique. A number of the most disturbing symptoms of menopause can be regulated by mind conditioning and when you practice deep breathing, you can control the symptoms so they do not affect you as much.

- Proper Diet: Already expressed in the previous section of this book, equipping your diet with the right vitamins and nutrients is essential because there are certain substances that you may obtain from food. Instead of taking supplements, you can obtain them from natural sources, by carefully planning your diet. Food, remember, is fuel for the body and when supply yourself with enough of what it needs, you are giving it a better chance of protecting itself. Observing proper nutrition gives a generalized healthy well-being to anyone and even more so to a woman who is in her menopause years.

- Massage: Stress is known to exacerbate all kinds of conditions, even menopause symptoms. When you are dealing with stress, everything else will be so much harder to deal with. Getting an appointment with a massage therapist on a regular basis will help you deal with this. Massage will help you deal with menopause by increasing your blood circulation and flushing toxins out of your body, so that you feel more relaxed and at ease.

- Chiropractic Care: Most people associate Chiropractors only with back pain, but regular Chiropractic care can keep every system in your body working at its highest potential. A Chiropractor's philosophy is to heal the body without medication, by keeping your spine and nervous system in proper alignment so your brain is able to communicate correctly with all the organs and systems throughout your body.

Think of it this way your brain is connected to everything in your body through your nervous system, just like with an electric cord attached to an electric device. If there is an obstruction or a "kink" in the wire the device will not work correctly. This is also true with in your body, if your spine is out of alignment it can put pressure or cause a "kink" in a nerve that runs through your body, therefore causing a lack of proper communication to your brain.

If your brain is able to communicate with the rest of your body at 100% you will notice that symptoms such as; headaches, hot flashes, depression and night sweats may decrease naturally without the use of medications.

- Proper Clothing. Hot flashes are excruciatingly difficult to bear and one of the best ways to deal with it would be to dress appropriately. Dress in light material so that your body can breathe well and perspiration is allowed to escape properly through your clothing. You can also try to cool yourself by having consuming cold drinks, taking cold showers and staying in sufficiently cooled venues.

- Rest and Sleep. Make sure to get enough rest and sleep on a daily basis. Avoid stress and other stimulants such as coffee and alcohol, which will only bring you more discomfort. Hot flashes may manifest as "night sweats" so staying up all night is going to be more difficult to bear. Give yourself enough rest and sleep so that your body will be strong enough to deal with the symptoms of menopause.

- Quit Smoking. If you are a smoker and you have incessantly failed on quitting the habit, now is the right time to do it. Smoking is generally bad habit, because it can cause all kinds of problems. It can increase the risk of heart disease, osteoporosis, stroke and cancer.

As the body's production of vital female hormones such as estrogen comes to a halt during menopause, a woman will start to experience a wide array of physical and emotional symptoms caused by hormonal imbalance. It may seem overwhelming and disheartening to know that this hormonal rollercoaster of highs and lows (or fluctuations) will happen for a couple of years or even more. However, knowing what they are and understanding why they are happening will help alleviate some of these negative feelings. It will also help when considering options in managing these symptoms.

Below are the three most common signs of menopause: **Hot Flashes** Hot flashes are the most popular symptoms among women. Oftentimes, when asked what menopause is, people will often think of hot flashes. What are hot flashes exactly and why are they called such?

A sudden temporary spike in the body temperature due to hormone fluctuations is responsible for hot flashes. When this happens, the body's external temperature surges rapidly and then slowly goes back to normal. These flashes are often accompanied by flushing, sweating and at times, light headedness. Duration and frequency varies and can happen anytime of the day. When they happen at night, they are often called night sweats.

How do you know that you are experiencing hot flashes? If you answered "yes" to most of the questions below, chances are you are having hot flashes:

- Do you experience a sudden intense feeling of heat emanating from all parts of your body especially on the neck, arms and torso?

- Do you notice your face reddening or flushing?

- Do you feel your heart suddenly palpitating?

- Does your pulse quicken?

- Do you experience perspiration and chills?

- Do you suffer from dizziness, nausea, and, at times, headaches?

Vaginal Dryness Many women are embarrassed about it but this is a normal occurrence during the transition years to menopause. It was revealed in studies that about40% to 60% of women experience vaginal dryness during the perimenopause stage. This is primarily due to the continuously dwindling levels of estrogen in a woman's body.

The blood vessels in a woman's vaginal wall secrete a clear fluid providing natural lubrication. Vaginal dryness or atrophic vaginitis happens when there is lack of adequate moisture in the vaginal area.

Go over the questions below and find out if you are experiencing vaginal dryness:

- Do you suffer from itching?

- Has intercourse been painful lately? And do you experience light bleeding after?

- Do you experience a burning and stinging sensation down there?

- Do you feel an unexplained pressure on your vaginal area?

- Do you feel discomfort when wearing tight pants?

- Are you urinating more frequently than usual?

- Do you experience general discomfort in the vaginal area?

Mood Swings The seemingly unending fluctuations of hormones also have a tremendous effect on a woman's emotions and moods. And just like her hormone levels, her moods also go through peaks and lows, oftentimes abrupt and extreme. It is like a pendulum that swings rapidly almost to the point of going out of control.

Estrogen influences the production of serotonin which is commonly known as the mood chemical. It is a chemical produced by the body that acts as a neurotransmitter. It is popularly known to affect and balance a person's moods and emotions. Other symptoms of transition to menopause like night sweats, fatigue and hot flashes can also cause irritability and mood swings. These triggers however, are still caused by hormonal imbalance.

Below are some questions you can go through to assess if you are experiencing mood swings:

- Do you feel an unexplainable surge of emotions like sadness, anger, and depression?

- Do you find yourself lacking the drive or motivation to go through the day?

- Have you been impatient, aggressive and irritable lately towards things that you normally don't pay much attention to?

- Are you feeling more and more stressed lately?

- Do you experience bouts of anxiety and nervousness and doesn't know why?

- Have you been feeling more and more melancholic lately?

No Sex Drive Probably the most discomforting, sensitive, and embarrassing symptom of perimenopause for most women is the loss of libido. Many women are not comfortable talking about it because they don't want to be deemed inadequate. Not only have they lost the ability to reproduce, they now also find themselves unable to satisfy their partner's sexual desires. This, however, is normal and many women going through menopause experience this.

During this time, many women lose interest in engaging in sexual activities. They may find themselves having less and less sexual feelings toward their partners. Other factors that may contribute to low or no sex drive are vaginal dryness and irritation, as well as mood swings. Again, these are all due to the dwindling presence of female sex hormones in a woman's body.

Below are some questions you can go through to find if you are losing your libido:

- Have you been feeling less and less attracted, sexually, to your partner?

- Do you find yourself becoming less responsive to things that used to stimulate you sexually?

- Do you often think of sex now as more of a chore than an activity that you enjoy?

- Do you lack energy for sex?

The four highlighted symptoms are the most common among many women. The list of symptoms however, is much longer. Here are some of them. Do take note that the symptoms are not limited to those that are listed below:

- Hair loss

- Fatigue

- Memory lapses

- Bloating

- Digestive problems

- Bone loss or osteoporosis

- Incontinence or other urinary health issues

- Weight gain

- Sleep disorders like insomnia

- Irregular periods

Knowing the pains and discomfort that come with the perimenopause years will equip women, especially the younger ones, with knowledge on how to deal with these issues when the time comes. As early as their 30s, women can start looking into possible lifestyle changes to diminish the symptoms that hormonal imbalance will bring upon their bodies.

Chapter 3: Changing Your Lifestyle

Your lifestyle can affect the intensity of the symptoms of menopause. Menopausal woman will benefit from staying active, because they will be able to deal with the symptoms associated with menopause more easily. The following are some of things you can do which have scientific significance. An even more natural approach to the condition that takes away the need for medicines and treatments will involve making a lifestyle change and incorporating these activities into your daily routine.

Here is a list of some activities and habits you can incorporate into your everyday life:

- Exercises: It does not matter type of exercising you do; it will help make your life better as you go through the stages of menopause. Exercising will strengthen your cardiovascular system, improve your mood by releasing endorphins, protect your body against diabetes, as well as osteoporosis by strengthen your bones and muscles.

If you have been an avid health buff throughout your life continue your normal routine even into your menopausal years. If you have never done any exercising through out your life, do not be threatened to start a new routine because it will be easy to get used to the activity once you get your groove and find a specific exercise you enjoy. There a number of different activities you can do: running, biking, dancing, swimming, aerobics and so many others. To find which on is best for you, try many different things until you find the activities you enjoy doing. When you find an exercise that is right for you commit to a regular routine so that you can truly see the great health benefits you will get from a consistent effort.

- Yoga: Yoga is not only a physical exercise it is an activity that can condition your mind as well. When you participate in yoga, you are able to increase your flexibility and you develop stronger muscles and bones in the process. Also, the meditative nature of yoga will help you deal with the mood swings associated with menopause. Menopausal women are easily irritated and annoyed so meditation will help to calm the nerves and ease the tension. A healthy mind and body is what you will get when you practice yoga. There are many different types of yoga classes you can join at your gym. Try them all until you find the one you like. You can also find exercise videos online that you can do at home, at youtube.com or you can purchase exercise dvds as well.

- Breathing Exercises: You will learn deep breathing techniques through your yoga instructor. Deep breathing is a very effective relaxation technique. A number of the most disturbing symptoms of menopause can be regulated by mind conditioning and when you practice deep breathing, you can control the symptoms so they do not affect you as much.

- Proper Diet: Already expressed in the previous section of this book, equipping your diet with the right vitamins and nutrients is essential because there are certain substances that you may obtain from food. Instead of taking supplements, you can obtain them from natural sources, by carefully planning your diet. Food, remember, is fuel for the body and when supply yourself with enough of what it needs, you are giving it a better chance of protecting itself. Observing proper nutrition gives a generalized healthy well-being to anyone and even more so to a woman who is in her menopause years.

- Massage: Stress is known to exacerbate all kinds of conditions, even menopause symptoms. When you are dealing with stress, everything else will be so much harder to deal with. Getting an appointment with a massage therapist on a regular basis will help you deal with this. Massage will help you deal with menopause by increasing your blood circulation and flushing toxins out of your body, so that you feel more relaxed and at ease.

- Chiropractic Care: Most people associate Chiropractors only with back pain, but regular Chiropractic care can keep every system in your body working at its highest potential. A Chiropractor's philosophy is to heal the body without medication, by keeping your spine and nervous system in proper alignment so your brain is able to communicate correctly with all the organs and systems throughout your body.

Think of it this way your brain is connected to everything in your body through your nervous system, just like with an electric cord attached to an electric device. If there is an obstruction or a "kink" in the wire the device will not work correctly. This is also true with in your body, if your spine is out of alignment it can put pressure or cause a "kink" in a nerve that runs through your body, therefore causing a lack of proper communication to your brain.

If your brain is able to communicate with the rest of your body at 100% you will notice that symptoms such as; headaches, hot flashes, depression and night sweats may decrease naturally without the use of medications.

- Proper Clothing. Hot flashes are excruciatingly difficult to bear and one of the best ways to deal with it would be to dress appropriately. Dress in light material so that your body can breathe well and perspiration is allowed to escape properly through your clothing. You can also try to cool yourself by having consuming cold drinks, taking cold showers and staying in sufficiently cooled venues.

- Rest and Sleep. Make sure to get enough rest and sleep on a daily basis. Avoid stress and other stimulants such as coffee and alcohol, which will only bring you more discomfort. Hot flashes may manifest as "night sweats" so staying up all night is going to be more difficult to bear. Give yourself enough rest and sleep so that your body will be strong enough to deal with the symptoms of menopause.

- Quit Smoking. If you are a smoker and you have incessantly failed on quitting the habit, now is the right time to do it. Smoking is generally bad habit, because it can cause all kinds of problems. It can increase the risk of heat disease, osteoporosis, stroke and cancer.

As the body's production of vital female hormones such as estrogen comes to a halt during menopause, a woman will start to experience a wide array of physical and emotional symptoms caused by hormonal imbalance. It may seem overwhelming and disheartening to know that this hormonal rollercoaster of highs and lows (or fluctuations) will happen for a couple of years or even more. However, knowing what they are and understanding why they are happening will help alleviate some of these negative feelings. It will also help when considering options in managing these symptoms.

Below are the three most common signs of menopause: **Hot Flashes** Hot flashes are the most popular symptoms among women. Oftentimes, when asked what menopause is, people will often think of hot flashes. What are hot flashes exactly and why are they called such?

A sudden temporary spike in the body temperature due to hormone fluctuations is responsible for hot flashes. When this happens, the body's external temperature surges rapidly and then slowly goes back to normal. These flashes are often accompanied by flushing, sweating and at times, light headedness. Duration and frequency varies and can happen anytime of the day. When they happen at night, they are often called night sweats.

How do you know that you are experiencing hot flashes? If you answered "yes" to most of the questions below, chances are you are having hot flashes:

- Do you experience a sudden intense feeling of heat emanating from all parts of your body especially on the neck, arms and torso?

- Do you notice your face reddening or flushing?
- Do you feel your heart suddenly palpitating?
- Does your pulse quicken?
- Do you experience perspiration and chills?
- Do you suffer from dizziness, nausea, and, at times, headaches?

Vaginal Dryness Many women are embarrassed about it but this is a normal occurrence during the transition years to menopause. It was revealed in studies that about40% to 60% of women experience vaginal dryness during the perimenopause stage. This is primarily due to the continuously dwindling levels of estrogen in a woman's body.

The blood vessels in a woman's vaginal wall secrete a clear fluid providing natural lubrication. Vaginal dryness or atrophic vaginitis happens when there is lack of adequate moisture in the vaginal area.

Go over the questions below and find out if you are experiencing vaginal dryness:

- Do you suffer from itching?

- Has intercourse been painful lately? And do you experience light bleeding after?

- Do you experience a burning and stinging sensation down there?

- Do you feel an unexplained pressure on your vaginal area?

- Do you feel discomfort when wearing tight pants?

- Are you urinating more frequently than usual?

- Do you experience general discomfort in the vaginal area?

Mood Swings The seemingly unending fluctuations of hormones also have a tremendous effect on a woman's emotions and moods. And just like her hormone levels, her moods also go through peaks and lows, oftentimes abrupt and extreme. It is like a pendulum that swings rapidly almost to the point of going out of control.

Estrogen influences the production of serotonin which is commonly known as the mood chemical. It is a chemical produced by the body that acts as a neurotransmitter. It is popularly known to affect and balance a person's moods and emotions. Other symptoms of transition to menopause like night sweats, fatigue and hot flashes can also cause irritability and mood swings. These triggers however, are still caused by hormonal imbalance.

Below are some questions you can go through to assess if you are experiencing mood swings:

- Do you feel an unexplainable surge of emotions like sadness, anger, and depression?
- Do you find yourself lacking the drive or motivation to go through the day?
- Have you been impatient, aggressive and irritable lately towards things that you normally don't pay much attention to?
- Are you feeling more and more stressed lately?
- Do you experience bouts of anxiety and nervousness and doesn't know why?
- Have you been feeling more and more melancholic lately?

No Sex Drive Probably the most discomforting, sensitive, and embarrassing symptom of perimenopause for most women is the loss of libido. Many women are not comfortable talking about it because they don't want to be deemed inadequate. Not only have they lost the ability to reproduce, they now also find themselves unable to satisfy their partner's sexual desires. This, however, is normal and many women going through menopause experience this.

During this time, many women lose interest in engaging in sexual activities. They may find themselves having less and less sexual feelings toward their partners. Other factors that may contribute to low or no sex drive are vaginal dryness and irritation, as well as mood swings. Again, these are all due to the dwindling presence of female sex hormones in a woman's body.

Below are some questions you can go through to find if you are losing your libido:

- Have you been feeling less and less attracted, sexually, to your partner?
- Do you find yourself becoming less responsive to things that used to stimulate you sexually?
- Do you often think of sex now as more of a chore than an activity that you enjoy?
- Do you lack energy for sex?

The four highlighted symptoms are the most common among many women. The list of symptoms however, is much longer. Here are some of them. Do take note that the symptoms are not limited to those that are listed below:

- Hair loss
- Fatigue
- Memory lapses
- Bloating
- Digestive problems
- Bone loss or osteoporosis
- Incontinence or other urinary health issues
- Weight gain
- Sleep disorders like insomnia
- Irregular periods

Knowing the pains and discomfort that come with the perimenopause years will equip women, especially the younger ones, with knowledge on how to deal with these issues when the time comes. As early as their 30s, women can start looking into possible lifestyle changes to diminish the symptoms that hormonal imbalance will bring upon their bodies.

Chapter 4: Facing Menopause Head-On with medical treatments.

While it is encouraged that everyone tries to deal with menopause naturally, know that that there are medical treatments and medications available. All of these treatments are proven to help relieve menopausal symptoms, but come with very high risks of developing things like cancer and strokes.

1. HRT (Hormone Replacement Therapy)
Hormone Replacement Therapy or simply, Hormone Therapy makes use of the combination of progestin and estrogen. It is ideal for women with or without a uterus because it can manage hot flashes, prevent bone loss and avoid fractures that are osteoporotic in nature. When the hormone levels are declining, the symptoms mentioned will become a big issue. Understand

that your body is exhibiting these changes because of hormone imbalances.

It is available in various forms: transdermal (patch or spray) and pill—the transdermal route being the safest because it does not go through the liver, but despite its capacity and function, it is used in moderation given the number of risks involved and it should only be used for a short period of time, using a relatively low dosage. This is preferred as an alternative treatment and never the first resort.

Risks and Side-effects: - It can increase the risk of blood clots and strokes.

- It can cause tenderness of breast and can even increase the risk of developing breast cancer - It can increase the risk of developing endometrial cancer, which is the cancer of the lining of the uterus - It can cause excessive weight gain and mood changes - It can cause nausea and headaches

2. Bio identical Hormones

The term "biogenetical" suggest that they are chemically identical to natural hormones. These are medications that contain hormones that are of the same formula as those that are naturally synthesized by the body. Derived from naturally-occurring plant products, these hormones are created in a laboratory.

Tibolone, an example of a bioidentical hormone may be taken in combination with or as an alternative to HRT. It can help a woman deal with symptoms such as improving sex drive and controlling hot flashes and night sweats.

Risks and Side-effects: - While there are some formulations that are FDA-approved and are safe for use, as they are manufactured by drug companies, there are some preparations that are manufactured in compounded pharmacies which are not approved and therefore not safe for use.

- While there is no reported danger to the transdermal form of bio identical hormones, there is no conclusive study that will confirm its safety. Its safety and long-term effects are not yet proven, so using it still come with risks.

- The use of Tibolone comes with an accompanying risk of developing breast cancer, uterine cancer and strokes. It is also not a suitable hormone treatment for women over the age of 60 years old.

3. Birth Control Pills

Oral contraceptive pills may be used as hormone therapy and it is usually prescribed for premenopausal woman who are experiencing irregular bleeding. As long as it has been found certain that the abnormal bleeding episodes are not being caused by any other problem, oral contraceptives can be given in combination with hormone therapies to bring some regularity to the menstrual cycle and can relieve hot flashes.

Risks and Side-effects: - It can cause high blood pressure, heart attacks, strokes and blood clots - It can cause weight gain

4. Estrogen Therapy, Creams and Tablets

Local (vaginal) hormone and non-hormone treatments are medications that are applied directly on the vagina. They are rings, creams and tablets that contain estrogen and are like hormone replacement treatments. Within this category, vaginal moisturizers could be included because they are designed to give some relief, especially for vaginal dryness during sexual intercourse.

Note: You should avoid vaginal lubricants with glycerin content because it can cause burning and discomfort. As much as possible, choose water-based products that are more delicate on the skin.

Risks and Side-effects: - May cause skin irritations - Estradiol, a major component of vaginal creams increase the risk of endometrial hyperplasia that can cause cancer of the lining of the uterus - Increased risk of stroke - Can cause nausea and vomiting - Can cause withdrawal bleeding

5. Selective Estrogen Receptor Modulators (SERMSs)

Raloxifene and tamoxifne are the most commonly prescribed SERMs and they are composed of phytoserms or drugs which are synthesized from various botanical sources. They are either agonists or antagonists of estrogen found all over the body.

Raloxifene is an agonist to bone and lipid changes; and an antagonist to endometrium and breast changes in the body. It is also capable of preventing vertebral fractures cause by osteoporosis.

Risks and Side-effects:

- It can increase the intensity of hot flashes

Surviving the Menopausal Years

Surviving Menopause may seem like a challenge, but you will get through this time in your life. You can go about it on your own naturally or you can see about working things out with your doctor. Whether you choose to go about it naturally or with the help of medicine, you need to confirm that you are indeed menopausal, so visiting your doctor for proper diagnosis will help.

Equip yourself with the following before you see the doctor: 1. Make sure you have made a list of your symptoms and have properly recorded specific details about them. How frequent are they? How severe are they felt? How long do the attacks go? What are the triggers?

2. Make a note of all the medications (natural or commercially sold) that you have taken, to relieve yourself of the symptoms of that you feel. How long have you been taking them? How often do you take them? What dosage or quantity do you consume? What are the effects of these medications on you?

3. Prepare a list of questions to ask the physician. You may think you won't forget but people usually do, once they are in the office, so take them down and share your concerns to your doctor.

4. Have a notebook with you so that you can conveniently take down information and instructions that your doctor will impart with you during the session. A lot will be talked about and you may not remember some of the details so it is best to take down notes so that you can refer to them later.

5. Inquire about what you can use that would help with your experience: books, websites, seminars, groups, alternative therapies and so forth. While these referrals can be obtained all around it is still best that you consult a well-informed expert about this because they can give you better guidance.

6. Expect the doctor to make inquiries about you and your condition. Be truthful about every aspect of your condition so that the doctor could make a better assessment of your case.

7. Do you your own research on the treatments your doctor may prescribe. Just because it is a medication prescribed by a doctor does not mean it is completely safe. Find out what the risks

involved are and if the treatment is right for you. Equip yourself with knowledge so that you can know what questions to ask your doctor.

The best advice we could give you is to eat whole foods that are not processed and exist in nature, naturally. Stick to your fruits, veggies, lean meats and fish. Don't fall for the gimmicky processed canned foods, dinners in a bag, veggies you cook in a bag in the microwave, rice with seasonings in a box, cereals, dairy, milk, breads, yogurt etc. that claim to be healthy with certain "added vitamins". Read the labels on everything before you buy it, know what is in your food.

Also, try to eat organically grown fruits and vegetables there are many harmful chemicals that are put in and on foods during farming and processing. It is advised to eat organically grown fruits and vegetables because there are no pesticides. Some pesticides that are put on the fruits and vegetables to kill bugs are also harmful to humans. They are called neurotoxins and they disrupt brain function and cause other problems within the body. It is important to research the foods and products you use on a daily basis to see what chemicals you are putting into your body. Check the label on the meats as well, especially chicken and eggs. You want to buy the ones that say no added hormones or antibiotics, grass feed, or range free.

Now we will list different vitamins and minerals that are a good source to incorporate into your diet. We will tell you why these vitamins are good for menopausal women and what foods contain them naturally.

1. Omega 3 Fatty Acids are one of the best things you can incorporate into your diet. You will find omega 3's in foods like wild caught fish; salmon and halibut, extra virgin olive oil, flaxseeds, walnuts, pumpkin seeds, Brussel sprouts and cauliflower. Omega 3's has anti-inflammatory

properties and are used all throughout your body.

2. Omega 6 Fatty Acids work in conjunction with omega 3's and are best when they are kept in balance with your omega 3 intake. In most Americans' diet we consume too much omega 6's and not enough omega 3's. Omega 6's aid in the production of hormones, but they have an inflammatory effect if intake is too high. Omega 6's can be found in many foods from chicken, beef, pork, dairy, breakfast cereals, soy beans, peppers, onions, potatoes, fast foods and prepackaged snacks.

Here is a good rule: most animal fats have omega 6, if the fat is solid at room temperature then it is most likely an omega 6. For example, the marbling in a steak at room temperature is not liquid it is a solid and blends in with the constancy of the meat. Chicken fat is another omega 6 which you will see that is mostly solid at room temperature.

Fish is different because it lives in cold water environments and can not have fat solidifying when the it's swimming around. So, the fat must remain liquid at cooler temperatures this is an example of omega 3's.

So, how do omega 3's and omega 6's work together? A four to one ratio of omega 6's to omega 3's, or two omegas 6's to one omega 3 is the common rule.

The fact of the matter is most Americans have a sixteen to one ratio of omega 6's to omega 3's, which is far too high omega 6. This can be the cause of many inflammatory conditions, such as, rheumatoid arthritis, psoriatic arthritis, lupus, osteoarthritis, asthma, common allergies, and most importantly can cause the overproduction of hormones, which play a significant role in menopausal symptoms. Remember omega 6's plays a role in hormone production. When these are not imbalance it can cause hormones to be produced in incorrect proportions causing; hot flashes, night sweats, mood swings, vaginal dryness, etc.

3. Calcium-Is important to bone health. During menopause your body starts to lose the ability to absorb calcium, so it is important to try to keep your calcium levels up.

Most people think of milk, yogurt, and cheese as a significant means to get their intake of calcium, but there are many other healthier choices that will be better for your body. Not only is milk high in fat, but it is not made how it used to be, it is now a processed food.

Today a lot of the milk industries get their milk from cows that have been given high doses of antibiotics and hormones, which can in turn end up in the milk you drink. This is especially bad for menopausal women, because it can disrupt their bodies ability to control its hormone levels. The key to being healthy during menopause is giving your body what it needs to balance your hormone level, and milk will do the opposite.

Here is a list of healthy foods that contain calcium: kale, bok choy, okra, collard greens, broccoli, figs, oranges, white beans, almonds.

4. Vitamin K-Eating foods that are high in Vitamin K can aid in the prevention of heart disease, osteoporosis, cancer and Alzheimer's disease. It is also linked to improving the look of dark circles under your eyes. The most common foods that have Vitamin K are dark green leafy vegetables like kale, turnip greens, spinach,

Swiss chard, and mustard greens. Surprisingly herbs like oregano, basil, parsley, cilantro, and coriander are also high in Vitamin K. (If you are considering taking Vitamin K supplements speak to your doctor first.)

5. Vitamin D-Is essential for your bodies ability to absorb nutrients like calcium and vitamin k.

Vitamin D works together with Vitamin K and Calcium to help keep your bones healthy. It has also been linked to promoting healthy brain function later in life. Your body makes Vitamin D naturally through being exposed to sunlight. Although it is advised to go in the sun a little each day too much UV Rays can be harmful. So limit yourself to about 15 to 20 minutes each day. You can also get Vitamin D through your diet by eating foods like wild caught salmon, sardines, white button or Portobello mushrooms, and eggs. (Consult with your doctor of how long you should be exposed to the sun light. If you are considering taking Vitamin D supplements speak to your doctor first.)

6. Fiber-A diet high in fiber is known to keep your digestive tract healthy, which is essential in giving your body the best chance to absorb all of the vitamins and minerals you eat. People who have a diet rich in fiber are known to be at a healthier weight and have a lower risk of heart disease and intestinal problems. Introduce more fiber into your diet slowly or you may be spending some extra time in the bathroom.

Fiber is found in vegetables, fruits, and whole grains. Here is a list of some high fiber foods; lentils, artichokes, broccoli, black beans, brown rice, oatmeal, pears, apples, blackberries, and raspberries.

7. Vitamin E-Is shown to alleviate some of the symptoms associated with menopause such as hot flashes and vaginal dryness. It is also known to reduce the risk of heart disease.

Here is a list of foods high in vitamin e: Spinach, broccoli, mustard greens, tomatoes, avocados, pumpkin, squash, asparagus, mangos, kiwi, shrimp, trout, nuts, sunflower seeds, basil, paprika, olive oil,

8. Vitamin C-As you age your body slows down the production of the collagen in between the layers of your skin which is the cause of symptoms like vaginal dryness during menopause. Vitamin C can help to rebuild or slow the effects of the collagen break down therefore improving these symptoms.

Vitamin C is an antioxidant and is known to aid with boosting your immune system, which will help keep your body healthy during menopause.

Eat fruits and vegetables that are high in Vitamin C like; oranges, papayas, kiwis, guavas, strawberries, tomatoes, yellow peppers, cucumbers, broccoli, kale, and peas.

9. B Vitamins there are a variety of different types of B vitamins that you can easily include into your diet. With the exception of b12 which can only be found in meats. The best advice would be to eat the rainbow when it comes to vegetables. Including things like carrots, beets, green leafy vegetables, egg plant, squash, etc. Many of these include different types of b vitamins as well as other vitamins your body can utilize.

One-way vitamin b can help in the aging process is by reversing the deterioration of your muscles as you age. B Vitamins are also linked to healthy brain function and can help you feel more alert and clearheaded. They also increase metabolism and can help you stay a healthy weight and give you increased energy. B Vitamins also help to improve your skin and eye sight.

10. Magnesium-Is known to benefit menopausal women, because of it's role in bone health and mood stabilizing. Research has shown that magnesium is a natural sleep aid, reduces the occurrence of migraines, and also helps with anxiety. It also works together with calcium and vitamin d in keeping your bones healthy to prevent osteoporosis.

Here is a list of foods high in magnesium: collard greens, kale, spinach, avocados, black eyed peas, kidney beans, white beans, chickpeas, bananas, cashews, pine nuts and wild caught salmon

Talk to your doctor before adding any dietary supplements into your diet. Too much of anything is a bad thing and it is important to find balance. Everyone's body is different, pay attention to your body and how it reacts to certain foods, vitamins etc.

Now that you are aware of the mechanisms behind menopause, its different stages, and its long list of symptoms, the next step is for you to decide how you will manage these symptoms for you to be able to continue to enjoy life until your prime years. You should not be a slave to the pains and discomforts of your perimenopause phase. You don't have to wait it out until the symptoms go away. You can take charge of your body and use the knowledge that you have about menopause, to create a course of action that will most suit your body and your lifestyle.

There are five ways to manage perimenopause symptoms. The first option is to go the hormonal route. The second is choosing no hormonal medication. The third option is the natural way. The third option has three choices under it.

Going Hormonal Hormone Replacement Therapy or HRT is a popular and controversial way to manage the symptoms of menopause. The therapy's ultimate purpose is to replace the hormones that are no longer produced by a woman's body namely, estrogen and progesterone. There are two types of HRT. The first one is Estrogen Replacement Therapy and the second one is a combination of both hormones.

There are many ways to get these replacement hormones inside a woman's body. The most common is the estrogen pill. It is the top choice because it is convenient, inexpensive and very easy to administer. Estrogen can also be administered by using a patch. This is best for women who have the tendency to forget taking their estrogen pills on a daily basis. The patch is only applied about once or twice a week. Patches though may fall off especially during rigorous activities. Estrogen can also come in forms of creams or gels. They are often applied once or twice daily. These are however not regulated by FDA therefore, were not tested for safety. Estrogen can also be delivered via a hypodermic needle. Injections however are not widely used in the US. They are not convenient and usually require a visit to the doctor to administer the hormones. There are also estrogen vaginal creams available which are often used to manage vaginal dryness. Some hormones are also administered by inserting estrogen pellets under the skin. This process is not too popular as this also requires a visit to the doctor.

No hormonal There are also medications available that can combat and alleviate menopausal symptoms. Many can be taken orally and they don't alter the body's hormone levels.

Some antidepressants were found to be effective in elevating the body's serotonin which helps treat hot flashes and mood swings. Examples of these antidepressant medications are paroxetine, fluoxetine, and venlafaxine. Nonetheless, as much as these medications are effective, they also have side effects like dry mouth, constipation, nausea, insomnia and headaches.

Anti-seizure medication like Gabapentin is also used to reduce hot flashes.

High blood pressure medication clonidine is also another popular no hormonal medication that helps reduce hot flashes. It has the same effects as the antidepressants sans the mood enhancement part.

There are also vitamin supplements that can be taken to help alleviate the frequency of hot flashes. These are Magnesium and Vitamins E and B.

Going All Natural Though some women may consider using hormones or medication effective in combating the symptoms of the perimenopause stage, there are those who chose to counteract the effects of hormonal imbalance the natural way.

Oriental Medicine Alternative medicine like acupuncture is believed to ease hot flashes and other menopausal discomforts. Developed in Asia, this treatment uses very thin needles to activate the flow of vital life force energy in the body. The needles are inserted under the skin to relieve pain and enhance the body's well-being.

Acupressure is another practice that is also gaining popularity. Instead of needles, this technique uses finger point pressure. The pressure points, when activated are believed to release tension, ease pain and enhance the circulation of oxygen and nutrients in the body.

Herbs Use of herbal remedies is also gaining popularity among women who wish to manage their menopausal symptoms the natural way.

Some examples of these are licorice and ginseng. Others include red clover and black cohosh (a plant native to North America). The downside of using herbal remedies is that they are often not regulated by the FDA and some may contain toxins that might bring more harm to the body. For example, further studies of the effect of black cohosh showed that it can cause high liver toxicity. Therefore, it is best to consult first with a trained herbalist or a doctor before dabbing into these herbal remedies.

Yoga and Meditation Meditation is a practice that has been used for hundreds of years to calm the body, mind, and spirit. When meditating, a person trains the mind to focus the energy on certain body parts to receive healing. It helps lower the blood pressure and regulate breathing and heartbeat. It can also help improve the immune system. Meditation also trains the mind to rid itself of negative thoughts thus alleviating depression which can also be brought about by hormonal imbalance.

Yoga is another practice that can provide physical, mental, and emotional benefits to women going through the premenopausal phase. It is an ancient discipline that aims to transform and unite the body, mind and spirit through meditation and the practice of different poses or asana. During the practice of exercise, the body is trained to hold poses while focusing on the breath. This in turn helps calm the body including one's heartbeat and pulse. The poses can also include some hip openers and stretches that can help strengthen the vaginal wall and pelvis. There are also poses that help maintain core strength and joint and muscle flexibility, making the body more limber and less prone to injuries.

Lifestyle Changes: As a person ages, the body also ages. There will come a point when a change in lifestyle will become necessary not because the person is feeling his or her age but simply because the body can no longer take all the partying and sleepless nights.

Maintaining a healthy lifestyle can be beneficial in the long run especially for women. Once they hit the menopausal stage, they will reap the fruits of the lifestyle choices they made when they were younger.

Here some lifestyle changes that can help women during their menopausal phase:

- Kick the habit. If you're smoking, now is the time to give it up. Smoking has bad effects not just on the lungs but also on the bones, heart, and blood pressure too.

- Watch the weight. You don't have to be skinny. You just need to keep a healthy body weight, one that is fit for your age.

- Keep it cool. Keep your room cool. Choose clothes that are airy and those that don't trap heat. If the temperature is cold where you are at, dress in layers so that it will be easier for you to remove them when hot flashes occur.

- Relax. Lessen your stress level as much and as often as you can.

- Laugh and smile more. Maintain a positive outlook as much as you can.

- Maintain a healthy relationship with your friends and families. They will be your best support group when times get rough.

Given the numerous options available to battle the discomforts that come with the menopausal stage, it would be very tempting to select the easiest and most convenient way. Keep in mind though that in the end, your decision will depend on what your body tells you it needs. Seek out the help of professionals. Know all your options but be very critical about them. Know all the pros and the cons. Write down what works for you and what doesn't. Research and ask questions. Weigh them carefully. And finally, listen to your body.

Chapter 5: What You Eat Matters

Nutrition during the menopausal years plays a crucial role in combating the discomfort and symptoms that come with it. Your body uses whatever you feed it when adapting to the changes that is happening inside it. If you are feeding it poorly, then, chances are, you are not doing yourself any favor. Your body needs all the support it can get and good nutrition is one of them.

Go Easy On...

Fats. Cut down on saturated fats. Say goodbye to French fries, ice cream and full cream milk. Lessen your intake of trans fats which are often found in baked goods (yes, those cakes and yummy desserts). They increase the risk of heart disease and high blood pressure.

Salt and Sugar. Use them in moderation. Too much sugar can increase the likelihood of diabetes. Sugar is also a culprit for weight gains. Too much sodium on the other hand has been linked to high blood pressure as well as some urinary health problems.

Alcohol. Limit the margaritas and mojitos. A glass or two is enough. Binge drinking days are over. Too much alcohol can hasten bone loss. Plus, not to mention the damages it can cause to your liver.

Fizzy drinks. Yes, soda and other carbonated drinks can hamper calcium absorption. Eating all those dairy products and calcium-rich foods will go to waste if your body can't absorb them.

Spicy foods. These can make those hot flashes soar through the roof.

Coffee and tea. These are stimulants that can also add body heat and worsen hot flashes. They are also known to hinder body absorption of nutrients.

Focus More On...

Calcium. Keep your bones strong and healthy. Drink and eat two to four servings of dairy and food rich in calcium daily. Examples of food rich in calcium are sardines, salmon, broccoli and legumes. Calcium supplements are also available.

Iron. Eat about three servings of food rich in iron like red meat, green leafy vegetables, fish and poultry. Iron helps maintain a healthy immune system.

Fiber. Load up on fiber by eating foods like whole-grain breads, cereals, brown rice, pasta, fruits and vegetables. Fiber cleanses your body and helps it get rid of toxins.

During menopausal stage, it is important to maintain a balanced diet. Too much of anything is bad. Always keep your food intake in moderation. Read the labels of the food that you eat. Know what you are eating. Every time you eat, think of your body and how the food that you ingested will affect it. With this in mind, you will be more watchful of the food that you eat. Your body is your only ally so you have to be mindful of every food that it takes in. You are the only person responsible for its health and well-being.

Chapter 7: Exercise

It is important to stay active during menopause to help your body be as healthy as possible. Exercise not only keeps you at a healthy weight, but also increases levels of endorphins and serotonin in your brain. By increasing these levels you will experience an all over happier and more vibrant mood.

Here is a list of some exercise that can be great for women going through menopause:

2. Rhythmic Exercise is pretty much the same as dancing. Dancing helps make you feel better and helps you express your feelings through movements and beats. Rhythmic exercise is done by dancing along to a fast or slow tune. Dance along the beat of the song and express your

feelings and emotions while dancing. You may dance with some friends to boost your mood.

Rhythmic exercise not only helps you physically, but it also helps you mentally. Rhythmic exercises help improve flexibility and strength, improve posture and relieve pain. Aside from these, rhythmic exercises also help boost your energy, improve your mood and reduce depression. There are different kinds of rhythmic dancing, you may try ballroom, Zumba, Belly dancing, or even Hip Hop.

3. Walking or Jogging can be an easy way to incorporate exercise into your daily routine. Plan on going for a walk in the morning before or work, or in the evening after dinner. Thirty minutes to an hour every couple of days will be very beneficial in staying happy and healthy.

4. The best advice for working out is to join a gym. Most gyms offer a variety of aerobic classes that are fun and keep you active. Signing up for classes can also keep you in a routine of working out, because you have an obligation to be there. Plus you will meet new people and have fun!

Things That Will Keep You Healthy

Natural health practices are becoming more and more accepted. They are a better approach to curing the underlying causes of your problems. Rather than the medical treatments/medications that only mask your symptoms but don't treat the underlying causes.

1. Chiropractic Care-Chiropractors are mostly known for taking care of people with neck and back pain. Chiropractic care is so much more than that and has been shown to greatly improve the symptoms associated with menopause.

Chiropractic can best be described in this way. Your spinal cord is the center that relays messages sent from your brain through your spinal cord to your nervous system. Surrounding your spinal cord is a protective shield known as your spine and vertebrae. But what happens when your vertebrae are not in the correct place along your spine? This can happen during childbirth, after a car accident, after a big fall, or by sleeping in a damaging position just to name a few causes.

When your vertebrae are in misalignment they can pinch nerves that go to your organs, muscles and disrupt other vital functions throughout your body. This can affect many things from reproductive function to brain function. Chiropractic care is a safe way to treat menopause and menopausal symptoms. A Chiropractor will use different techniques to put the spine back in alignment so that your body can work at it's optimal level.

By releasing the tension off the nerves a Chiropractor can greatly improve your all over brain and nervous system function. By increasing brain function, you will notice a reduction in things like hot flashes, mood swings, weight gain, night sweats, irregular cycle, vaginal dryness, lowered sex drive, tiredness, dizziness, depression, anxiety, headaches and osteoporosis.

Protecting Yourself after Menopause

For most experts and health practitioners, menopause is the great time to keep women reminded to act and do something to prevent potential serious health diseases such as osteoporosis, breast cancer, cervical cancer and heart problems. Likewise, it is essential to have an annual physical check-up that includes several tests so you can have a heads-up on your health condition and what are your risks to get ill. Also, you may want to undergo gynecological tests such as breast exams, pelvic exams and pap smears. This can be also the best time to discuss with your doctor the medical history of your family so to make sure that you are provided with the right tests during and after menopause.

HEART HEALTH

Apparently, the leading cause of death across the United States is heart disease. Thus, adult women should have their cholesterol level check every five years even before menopause. This test along with blood pressure checking must be continuous after menopause. Other doctors recommend additional test such as blood tests, stress test or an ultrasound of the heart to further assess its overall function.

There are recent studies showing the correlation between high risk of heart disease and severe symptoms of menopause. The implication is women with severe symptoms can be at higher risk of heart disease. If you are experiencing extreme symptoms of menopause, talk with your doctor immediately to assess your heart's condition.

BONE MINERAL DENSITY TEST

The National Osteoporosis Foundation suggests that women who have higher risks of bone density should have regular bone mineral density test starting at their 50s. For those with low risk, they can wait until the age of 65. Some of the known risks are early or premature menopause, history of osteoporosis in the family, low body mass, tobacco use, history of medical conditions such as rheumatoid arthritis, some type of cancers, and hyperthyroidism. DEXA and ultrasound are two of the most common bone density tests that are bot invasive and out-patient procedures.

PELVIC EXAMS AND PAP SMEARS

These two can help you determine and early detect cervical cancer. The frequency of these tests depends on your risk level for cancer. For most women, every three years is sufficient. Check with your health care provider to see what applies to you.

BREAST EXAMS

This is the best time to get you started in getting mammogram if you haven't already done it. Screenings are advised to do every other year for women ages 50 to 74 years old. The American Cancer Society on the other hand stand with their recommendation of starting the annual screening as early as 40 years old. Other research says the frequency and timing of the mammogram is a decision that can be customized based on a woman's preference.

COLON CANCER SCREENING

Screening test for colon cancer such as colonoscopy is also highly advisable during menopause. Over the age of 50, it is the second leading cancer killer. Colonoscopy helps detect the cancer at an early stage however; most of us do not take advantage of this advantage.

Set an Appointment

All these tests may vary from one woman to another so it is best to consult your doctor first. Most likely, tour first appointment will be with your chosen gynecologist. And because appointments with the doctor are usually brief, prepare these things in advance;

Determine your symptoms - make a list of the symptoms you are experiencing and the frequency and severity of each symptoms.

List your medications - make a list of all the medication, vitamin supplements and herbs you are taking. Include the dosage and frequency as well.

Have someone accompany you-you will be given chunks of information and it can be difficult for you to remember all of those.

Notepad in handy - take a notepad or notebook with you so you can track the vital information of your every visit.

Get ready with your questions - list all the possible questions you would want to ask your doctor to avoid forgetting them. Some of the basic questions are the kind of tests you will need, the treatment options you have, how to relieve the symptoms and the alternative therapies applicable for you.

Moreover, expect your doctor to ask you questions such as when was the last time you had your last period, how do you think the symptoms worse, what bothers you in these symptoms and the like so get ready with your answers.

Conclusion

Menopause is not a disease. It is not a disorder but the symptoms involved with the condition make life difficult for some women. Menopause can be accompanied by physical, mental and emotional effects that are difficult to endure, so necessary treatments, remedies and natural management strategies become truly valuable.

Women can approach menopause naturally, performing certain remedies and utilizing natural solutions which will deal with their body changes. Some people choose to take care of menopause through medical treatments and medications—they may work in covering up the symptoms, but come with dangerous side affects such as developing cancer.

If you are going through menopause, understand that your body is going through changes that you will have to adjust to. It is so much more than the end of your period or menstruation. It is a new stage in your life of growth and realization. You have the power to get through this, menopause is not a bad thing, just a fact of life. All women go through this and in the end it is a beautiful thing. You will be even stronger than you were before this began. So, stay strong and take steps to keep your self healthy through diet and exercise. Although, the symptoms associated with menopause will make life more difficult, finding a balance through Yoga, herbal supplements and Chiropractic care can help tremendously. We hope that this book has helped you in this journey we call life.